HOW TO LOSE WEIGHT FAST

WEIGHT LOSS MOTIVATION & TIPS TO LOSE WEIGHT, BE HEALTHY IN 1 MONTH OR LESS THROUGH THE POWER OF PERSISTENCE

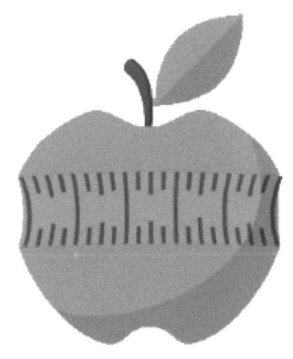

DAVID RODRIGUEZ

DEDICATION

This book is dedicated to my friends and family, who supported me in writing this book. I want to thank Karol Martinez, who was glad to accept an interview for this book. Thank you, for your honesty and willingness to share your story with us.

TABLE OF CONTENTS

INTRODUCTION

In today´s Western world, obesity is increasing at astonishing rates never before seen in our history. We have an abundance of unhealthy foods, and also our daily occupations bring ongoing stress to our busy lives, and unhealthy habits. All of these aspects of our modern society only have pushed obesity to record levels in America, and other civilized countries.

Millions of people simply give up when they are just getting started on their weight loss plans. Sometimes they even become paralyzed before starting, and do not do anything to lose weight and aim for a healthy lifestyle. These paralyzes or failed attempts can be related to fear of failure, wish for instant gratification, and other psychological issues that will find a root in one main topic: lack of persistence.

This book is going to help you identify the challenges that you can come across before or during your weight loss process that might spoil your success. It will also provide you with proven tips to accomplish shedding those pounds, and achieving success through the power that lies within every one of us: The power of persistence.

This book is going to increase your awareness of how the lack of persistence and other psychological concepts can keep making you fail to achieve your desired goals of a healthy weight and a healthy lifestyle.

I know of these challenges and tips because I am one of those people who, just like you, are struggling with overweight or obesity. This year, I found myself overweight, and one day I decided that I would get up and fight for my life and being healthy.

I am still not at my desired weight yet. My hope is by reading this book you will learn like me that there is a moment in this process where your body starts losing weight at its own rhythm. You need to go with the flow and keep following through to succeed.

I loved writing the book since I get the opportunity to share with you the tips that are going to help you succeed in your weight loss. I am excited that you are going to learn these tips in the following chapters.

The tips I wanted to share are worked for me or by the interesting people you will get to know in this book.

People of all social classes who struggle with persistence and some of them overweight and obesity have succeeded following the tips in this book.

You will meet Karol, a proud wife and mother of two, who when asked about the most difficult thing about weight loss replied: "Persistence is the most difficult aspect".

However, she will also tell us how she has successfully been able to lose 100 lbs in a short time.

I promise that if you finish the book and follow these tips complimenting them with a healthy diet and lifestyle, you are going to lose weight within the following 30 days. Not only that but also you will learn how to take ownership of your weight loss.

I promise you this short book is going to empower you by helping you discover that persistence, and determination we all have within us to achieve weight loss and a healthy lifestyle. First -as this is the challenge you are facing at this moment- but also your other important goals that you have set for yourself in life.

Don't keep failing with more attempts to lose weight due to lack of persistence and determination. I encourage you to push through those feelings of sadness that you have felt every time you have quit before.

Become the healthy person you have wanted to be all these years. Be the example for your family and friends when they look at you and say that achieving your dreams is possible when we make the decision to succeed. Be that happy person who has the confidence of knowing that you managed to lose weight, and you can manage whatever you want because you have uncovered the persistence within you.

Empower yourself right now with the power of persistence. It is proven. What you need to do is keep reading this powerful book. Take control of your weight and physical appearance, make it happen right now, enjoy the process and the new "you" that you will reveal.

START WITH YOUR "WHY"

"Why?" Every important single decision you make in life needs to be accompanied by a reason because this is going to give you the biggest motivation to stay on track, to be determined. This is a basic requirement, so to speak.

So, I present to you the most common reasons I consider important for losing weight and aiming for a healthy lifestyle in the lines below.

Prevent disease

First and foremost, you and me as humans have a survival instinct, we desire to stay alive. By losing weight, you are going to prevent diseases. I know that hundreds of diseases can occur from being overweight or fat. Let me introduce you to the most common diseases you will prevent/cure by shedding those pounds.

Heart disease

The number one spot, and the number one killer in the United States, and most of the Western world. High blood pressure comes along with it. I am sure no sane human would like to die from a stroke or heart attack; let me tell you, it is painful for you. Not only that, it is painful for your loved ones...

Let me share a personal story here that I hope illustrates the sadness of a real case of death from heart disease. I saw my grandmother die of a heart attack. I remember she was having a nice conversation one afternoon in 2006 with one of my aunts and I. When she stood up for a second to bring us some coffee from the kitchen, none of us, not even my grandma I suppose, knew what would happen in a split second later.

A heart attack struck her. She fell to the floor, the cup of coffee fell and broke in pieces. She started to vomit what she'd just eaten, she could not say a word. I remember her cute grandma face turn to a scared

4

expression, helpless, unable to defend herself from this killer. Her own heart could not resist to the pressure any longer. Sad but true, she died in front of two of her loved ones. She departed from this world suddenly.

Trust me that from my personal point of view, from that moment on, I knew I did not want to leave this world like that. Neither do I want this to happen to you nor your loved ones. You are taking one step towards your own improvement by reading this book.

Happier life

You may think, just like me when writing these lines, that being fit does not bring happiness in itself. That makes sense, but I also suggest you look at it this way…you may not be happier just by the mere act of being slim, but it can definitely make it easier. Let me give you one example, I love to learn with examples.

Say your chances to live longer and have more years with your family and friends increase exponentially as you avoid a list of hundreds of serious diseases. After a motorcycle accident, I realized that life is precious. Therefore, why not give the gift of life to enjoy with your friends and family. I can guarantee it is priceless when you think of it, even more when you experience situations close to death.

Here is a situation that I have seen happen to people who are obese, where it impacts their life and family. You are working a 9-5 job which means little time to enjoy time with your children. Add on top of that being obese, which limits what activities you can do with your children. I have seen that many parents cannot enjoy time with their kids fully because they do not have the ability to play with them. Instead, they have to sit down and watch them play.

This example may sound trivial, but to me it isn't, tell me, what is more, important than to be able to enjoy time with your family to your fullest?

One of our basic needs as humans is to feel accepted by our closest circle of peers, this can be your mom, your siblings, your spouse, feel free to fill the blank here. Do you need to believe that once you are on your way to losing more weight you are going to start to feel and look younger when you see yourself in the mirror? That is happening to me as I am writing this book. I am projecting that positive feeling to my family, which feels awesome. I want you to feel this way too.

Feel more energetic, creative, and sharp

We are all made of feelings. What is more positive than bringing more energy to your organism? It has happened to me on my weight loss path, my dear Padawan. And I believe that when a human being feels more daring and energetic, that can bring great abundance to their life.

Let me share with you my testimony. Before I started writing this book, around two months ago, I read and learned a list of ways to start a freelance career and eject my ass from the corporate world. This process has run parallel to my weight loss. I believe deep inside myself that the confidence I grew by shedding those 11 pounds in 3 months absolutely helped me to get up and quit my 9 to 5 job.

When you feel more energy than before by losing a few pounds, the world is at your feet. You will be boosting with confidence.

Need proof that energy increases? In the US, the National Heart, Lung, and Blood Institute (NHLBI) has made studies of the benefits of losing weight and having more energy is just one out of many.

Also, losing those pounds is going to sharpen your mind. You will notice your attention and memory improving, and what brings having a sharper brain? With a sharper brain comes a better performance in your daily activities such as working, exercising, studying or the daily buzz of taking care of your kids, and so on. As you can tell, everyone can benefit from a sharper mind.

In my case and I heard this happens to most people, weight loss has boosted my creativity as well. Shedding those pounds helped me remove a virtual cloud I had in my mind that made me think and act slower when I was heavier. Now everything seems less blurry. Bear in mind doctors state even if you lose just 5% of your body weight, all of these benefits will come to play. What can you do being more creative? Think about it. Maybe this will open a door of opportunity for a business idea that will bring you more wealth and abundance.

Build more self-confidence

There are a wealth of benefits that come from a healthy self-confidence. You will manage to tackle your fears with more ease, and other daily challenges too. It will help you maintain a positive mental attitude.

Your performance level will peak, and you will be a better achiever.

Imagine that you are an introvert, just like me. I have seen self-confidence help people feel more at ease during social interactions. This is a huge advantage on your side. Perhaps you are that guy who has been always afraid to take a step further and ask this pretty girl out. Or you are the lovely woman who is so afraid to ask her boss for a raise because you feel you do not deserve it.

You will feel stronger, as no matter what someone may tell you, the judgment of others is less important. Your self-confidence is internal, and it will not change based on external factors.

Self-confidence can and will bring more happiness to your life, as it is going to result in better relationships, your performance will go up. Let's be realistic here, a better performance can carry more money to your wallet as you can deliver more value to the world.

Personal satisfaction

Do you remember your high school graduation day? Giving birth to your child? A new promotion at work? The day when you bought that new house? That time when you bought the airplane ticket to a beautiful destination? The pleasurable feel of satisfaction that lies when you accomplish something that adds value to your existence? I hope just by reading above I can you bring back to that moment, bring you back to that sensation.

My friend, this is what I know you will experience again as you step on the scale and see those little numbers going down each time. I can tell you from experience that seeing just a couple of pounds less than last week on the scale gave me that type of internal joy. And the best part of that is you can get that feeling every week.

This is a similar to your gaining from a compound interest. The more joy you have in your life, the happier, the more productive, and lively you are. See what I mean?

Chapter summary

There you have it, the first part of the book. I hope you could squeeze all the juice out of this chapter. This part is truly important since as we may already know, you need to have a reason to go from point A to point B in your life. On your way to losing weight, otherwise, you may take or be lead to the wrong path, and we want all but the opposite.

Let me present a summary of the key points in this chapter we are closing now:

- You need a to have a "why" for losing weight

Here is an outline of reasons for losing those kilos:

- Prevent disease. Need I say more? Heart disease is at the top, and remember, this is an ugly way to say goodbye.

- Achieve a happier life

- Losing weight can help you be a more fulfilled human, and this can be shared with your friends and family.

- Feel more energy, be more creative, and sharp

All of these things can bring you bigger and better things. You will feel better than now, I guarantee.

Build more self-confidence and the world will be at your feet

Personal satisfaction

Do you remember the pleasurable feel of satisfaction that lies when you accomplish something that adds value to your existence? This is it. Losing weight and gaining life is priceless.

Let's move on to our next chapter. I really hope you are following along with me. We are going to dive deep into the psychological side of why most people give up to their weight loss fights.

Let me tell you, this is not you anymore; I sincerely believe that to be true as you are steps ahead already just by taking the initiative of purchasing this book.

However, the next section can motivate you to help other people who see their attempts at losing weight go down the drain without knowing why. If this were you not so long ago, it would also help you prevent this procrastination from happening again as you will be aware when it is knocking at your doorstep.

One old Chinese saying reads in Sun Tzu's The Art of War military treatise -a read I highly recommend by the way- that you must 'Know your enemy and know yourself, and you can fight a thousand battles without disaster. This is where I want to take you. I want you and your loved ones to win a thousand battles.

I would like to put the dots on the I''s here, see it as a disclosure: I'm not a psychologist, not that I want to become one. However, I want to help you on this book.

I am going to go over a few concepts you may notice when you are in your weight loss battle, and I believe I don't need to be a psychologist to write about these concepts. These are feelings, thoughts, which come to everyone at some point in their lives, and from my experience in my own weight loss fight, they were –and still are- frequent visitors. If you think your mind is winning over your goals for weight loss even after reading this book or any other book, if you are procrastinating this too much, please talk to your doctor.

This chapter may sound repetitive at times, but my hope is that you identify these bad guys when they want to come and sabotage your weight loss intentions.

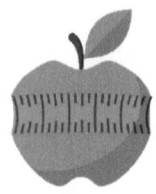

THE PSYCHOLOGICAL SIDE OF NOT BEING ABLE TO WIN THE WEIGHT LOSS BATTLE

First, I want to show you how new psychological concepts or problems have come to play for us human beings of the 21st century. The first one I wish to show you is…

Instant gratification

Maybe you have not heard of it, or probably you know about this from one of those Dr. Phil or Oprah TV shows. It's very simple. We have now turned into people who want things now, no matter what.

I believe technology plays an important role in this syndrome. We can contact people through an instant SMS or Whatsapp in our smartphone. We can order fast food just by picking up the phone and dialing the number. You name it. Many things are now so accessible than ever before. Credit cards help you buy that dress you want now, not tomorrow, now.

The disadvantage of this syndrome –besides the financial effects- is that in your case, when you want to lose weight. We are bombarded by so many products, plans, tv commercials that keep throwing at us stupid things like "lose 50 pounds in 3 days". Again, they take advantage of us 21st-century humans who want things done and ready as soon as possible. And even though what they promise is basically impossible, our subconscious mind stores the principle idea into our heads that we want to lose weight fast. Please, remember for your own good weight loss is one step at a time, these are baby steps, but also, don't think it is going to take forever.

Alongside the instant gratification, syndrome comes frustration, an old visitor since we were young.

Frustration

We want things now, and if we don't see immediate results, we feel frustrated to the point we feel like just giving up. Forgetting about our dreams and weight loss plans, and stopping by the McDonald's drive thru like we used to before.

You are more than this, and you can conquer this struggle. Just remember you need to take baby steps, one at a time. I suggest an old technique that worked for me whenever I feel frustrated…drink water, not fruit juice or soda, just plain bottled or tap water. I am pretty sure you will feel better, and the frustration will go away. Know your enemy when it's knocking at your door, is the key.

Another new problem that has come into play for us in the 21st century is modern distractions.

Modern distractions

For example, you planned to go to the gym or go outside to walk your dog, and suddenly before you head out or lace your shoes, you get a facebook message. You grab you phone, open facebook and spend unconsciously 10 or 15 minutes wandering in facebook reading the newsfeed. What comes next? When you are finished, you may think "I should go for that walk, but now it's getting dark, and I am tired, today was a busy day at the office."

You see? Nowadays it is so easy just to turn on your TV and watch that Netflix series instead of going to YouTube and searching for a home workout video, or taking a walk to the park. Don't fall for this trap. Just be brave and step to your door and get out. Walk your dog if you have one, will be good exercise for both of you. I can assure you the pain will stop immediately after you step out the door. You will overcome the mental barrier after that door. You can win this battle.

Complacent

Next, let's be aware that you may become complacent when it comes to weight loss too. You may believe that you are fine just being overweight. I am not saying you should hate yourself for not being slim but there is always a balance in life that can be attained.

However, what I would love to accomplish with this section is to shed a light of understanding that you and every person should always aim to be better, to grow, to go one step further.

You may say, "People love me even though I am fat" Or may even say "What if I lose weight, and all of a sudden people don't love me anymore as I am not going to be that funny fluffy guy (or girl)?". Well, that my friend is an excuse that is not going to help you anywhere in your process. I suggest you start believing people who really love you will still love you after you lose weight. Period. And again, you can always be better, and this is just the beginning.

Mediocrity

I want to put mediocrity as it can also be a bullet point in the list as one of the negative thoughts that may invade your mind if you allow it. It will probably come to your mind along with complacency. I picture them as a duo in this description of threats for your weight loss intents. I really hope not from now on.

Fatigue

When you are starting in on your weight loss process, or even in the middle of it, you may feel tired of doing this over and over. Sometimes it may seem like climbing an endless mountain, let me tell you, I have been there and done that. It may feel awful, and painful. Here is my piece of advice. Once a week, treat yourself. Maybe you want to buy an ice cream, eat a hot dog, or drink a Coke. Sounds good, right? I always have a day to treat myself with one of these things. After such hard work during those six days of the week, we all deserve it, don't you think? After all, you have worked out hard, cut your intake of calories throughout the week; you have sweated it out. Well done!

Also, sometimes it is only that you need to loosen up the effort, that you can lower the strength of your workout or diet. That is fine, every effort adds up, just as long as you keep going.

It would be different if you were to tell me you are tired even though you have not worked hard during the week, that you want to give up. I would suggest you drink more water, which gives more energy to your body. If even after that you still feel fatigued to a serious point that it never goes away, if you feel extreme exhaustion after physical activity or even after you sleep, if that were the case. I would suggest you visit your doctor. It may be a chronic fatigue syndrome. There is no medical explanation for this syndrome yet. The best you can do is talk to your doctor for an accurate diagnosis.

Fear of failure

I can think of the saying here by a mastermind of industry and business: "Whether you think you can, or you think you can't--you're right." Henry Ford

You have the power to keep things rolling; you are the one in charge. I like to think that whatever doesn't kill you makes you stronger. With my personal experience, there is no such thing as failure. What you need to do is stand up. If you fall nine times, stand up ten times.

You may think losing weight is too hard. That is up to you. Your body will lead you to the right pace; it will lead you to a balanced weight loss.

You may say, "I am not ready" I will do it whenever I am ready. The problem with that mindset is that if you wait for the perfect time to take action, you never will. Trust me. That's been proven by millions of people.

Financial reasons: "This is too expensive."

At some points, whether before starting your weight loss plan, even after you took action, you may think something like -"Oh no, this is going to be expensive".

You know what? It can be if you let it be, not necessarily. I have seen gyms charging huge sums of money for membership, monthly fees, all of that stuff. Also, there are millions of programs, memberships, seminars, diets, and so on for weight loss. The fact is this has become a huge industry since the 80s.

However, you don't need to pay for a gym membership to work out; you can work out at home following routines with YouTube videos, for example. You can find a healthy diet for low cost with a nutritionist. I mean, this doesn't have to be a big expense on your budget.

My take on this is there is nothing wrong with spending money for your weight loss. I see it as a great investment, same as if you were to invest in real estate, or in another business. You are investing in YOU. Health is a basic need for everybody. Why would you be stingy with yourself if you can afford this?

This may sound straightforward, but it is true. Would you prefer to spend money to prevent disease or to cure disease? There is a common consensus it will always be better that a person prevents disease instead of the second.

Chapter summary

We have covered eight mental barriers that are "enemies" of your weight loss. They are:

- Instant gratification
- Frustration
- Modern distractions
- Complacency
- Mediocrity
- Fatigue
- Fear of failure
- Financial reasons

I hope by now you can become more aware of them on a daily basis since they are extremely common.

Thank you for staying with me to this point of the journey. I hope you have learned something that motivates you to take action.

On the next chapter, I will tell you a story…My weight loss story. My weight loss is not finished yet, but I can tell you about how I have managed to cope with all the challenges and downsides that come to play so far.

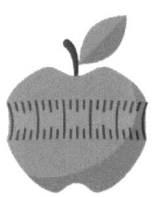

MY WEIGHT LOSS STORY

I am still 11 pounds from my goal when I started, but I know I am on the right track. Because, along the way I have learned –or even more, my body has taught me- how to lose weight at my rhythm. I am going to show how I have lost weight so far, this is not a cookie cutter solution, but it can help you with some tips for you through your own process.

I learned that drinking bottled water, even tap water (I am lucky enough to have drinkable water in my location) can help in a huge way to shed those pounds. I have been drinking a minimum of 1 liter (around 34 US ounces) every day religiously for the last four months. Let me tell you, it makes you feel less tired, and it helps your body eliminate more toxins, which leads to losing fat.

Do you hate the "taste" of water alone? What some people do is they put the juice of half a lime in it; it adds flavor to the equation. You may have heard this before, but it I will stress it again. Our body is made up of 80% of water, and it is a vital component we require to function properly. If possible, I would recommend you drink 2 liters every day this will help you see the most benefits.

Something I learned from a macrobiotic store: When you start with your weight loss plan, you should buy pills to cleanse your liver of all the toxins it accumulated through the years. It is a fact our liver has a way to cleaning itself when we are healthy. However, we have come to a point where we consume so much sugar, salt, alcohol, fatty foods, and chemicals. There is a list of components we eat almost every day that make our liver fat.

So, they recommended I should take a pill daily during the first two months. I did this and saw the difference. I think this is a great idea for anyone starting out. These pills are not expensive, they are around $8 USD in Amazon.com. I did not notice any side effects, again, ask your doctor for professional advice.

Talking about pills, I purchased a combo of pills for a ripped body composition, they are called GNC Pro Performance® AMP Ripped Vitapak® Program. They are a great product, you get 30 packs, one for each day, and they help you rid of excess liquid in your organism. There is one pill that helps boost your metabolism up to 12 times for up to one hour after exercise, another pill that helps you with carbohydrates metabolism.

One pill contains B-vitamins that are important for energy production; as a matter of fact, I felt more energetic at work, study and in my other daily tasks. I did not get any side effects with these pills either. They are made up of high quality ingredients, not bad chemicals. Having more energy can help you stick to your weight loss plan as I mentioned in the previous chapter. When you feel fatigued, you may want to give up. I highly recommend them. Please find a link at the end of the chapter if you want to see these pills for yourself.

Eat healthier: One thing I have done is read journals, expert columns about foods that are good for weight loss and also foods to avoid. I know I need to stay away from bread, fried food, overeating carbs, and sweetened foods. I just cut down the intake of these types of foods. I did not eliminate them all completely. For example, I would eat mashed potatoes once a week, or I could eat a candy bar once a week. In my case, I have not had to go to something extreme to lose weight. Additionally, eating healthier made me feel good, this sharpened my mind and body.

There are maybe millions of valid articles on the internet where you may find how to eat healthier. But more importantly, you should get advice from your doctor or nutritionist.

When it comes to exercise, let me share this story. I used to be skinny about six years ago; I started gaining weight as I started taking food supplements to do so. My problem was back then I gained around 10 lbs each year because I used to work in an office like millions of other people. So I worked in a seated position for 7 or 8 hours a day five days a week, and I did not take exercise very seriously. Months would pass with me not going to the gym, not eating healthy, nothing. These all added up to me becoming overweight.

About a year ago, I started going to the gym at least once a week. About four months ago, I started eating healthier, watching my diet, drinking plenty of water. I just did something every day. And I believe that little something added up to my weight loss. For instance, I would drink lots of water one day, on a different day I would cut down carbs. I tried my best to exercise for at least 90 minutes per week. You get me.

This may work for you, it helped me a lot. I used to drink alcohol every two weeks or so. I did this religiously for around three years. I would get drunk every time. Months ago, right when I started watching my diet too, I reduced my intake of alcoholic beverages. Since around five months ago, I have drank alcohol two to three times and just one beer each time. I deeply believe this will help you too. And as you may know, alcohol is mostly not good for your health. I say mostly because some benefits have been found to drinking a cup of wine every once in a while.

I have also quit smoking. We all know all the damage smoking tobacco has on our bodies. For me, I believe it was reducing my energy levels, and also it was causing hormonal imbalances, all of which are not good for a healthy body weight. I also used it as a way to deal with work stress, and instead of working out to release stress, I used to smoke.

I also paid for an abdomen reduction plan in esthetics clinic for the last four months. Although this may be regarded as unorthodox for my male readers, trust me, this helped me lose weight in a massive way. This plan helped me shed excess fat my body had and also to sculpt the abdomen area. Guys: don't fear this, don't fear losing your masculinity for going to one of these clinics. You will not lose anything. These placed are managed by professionals and remember this is yet another method to help you losing kilos.

Those were the things I did to lose weight. My goal is that you can use them as a blueprint for your plan. I believe a weight loss plan has different sides you need to look at, just like mine.

Challenges I have faced

I want to dedicate the second part of this chapter to my challenges in my weight loss process as well as the good times.

Work: Yep. Most of us have to do something for a living. In my case, I have had a job during this process. And there have been moments when I have felt too tired to eat healthy, too tired to work out. You get me. It can seem hard at times.

I want to encourage you to do something every day, even just a small step. What I have seen is the importance of being persistent with this goal, just like with other important goals we may have. Do not let work become an excuse for giving up on this. It is so simple to do just that. There will always be something who will support you on your excuses. There will always be someone backing up conformity.

People not caring: I know this may sound ridiculous, but I learned most people do not care about your intentions on losing weight. Your coworkers will just offer you to go to the fast food restaurant for lunch, as they did in the past, especially when you are just starting the process. They may think this idea of yours is not going to last, and one should not take it personally. Just remember only you have the power to achieve this and other goals. My suggestion would be to make the people around you aware of the plan and that you are serious. People who care about you will come to understand it at some point.

Frustration: I have felt frustrated sometimes as it is hard to get used to the idea of delaying gratification. Our culture teaches us that we should be asking to have things instantly and the easiest way possible. What a bad habit, especially when it makes us give up on important goals.

Sometimes I felt I was not making any progress. What a frustrating feeling. There was a moment when I felt like quitting. What kept me afloat was that I knew this was also part of the process. That there are "standby" moments when it seems nothing is happening and that all of our hard work makes no difference all. It is just a part of it.

Now I want to talk about the happy times.

Like I had mentioned earlier in the book, I noticed I had a sharper mind, and I had more energy at work and a better attitude towards every aspect of my life as I started losing weight. It pays off, and it is a great feeling when you step up on the scale and see the number is going down significantly. You feel pure satisfaction that you accomplished the mission you assigned for the week. Something I did was visualizing the weight I wanted to see on the scale each week. Visualizing my goal weight has helped me with my motivation.

Chapter 3 Summary

In this chapter, I wrote about my methods, challenges, and the good moments in my weight loss process.

Here is a breakdown of my methods:

- Drink water

- Liver cleansing pills

- GNC pills

- Eat more healthily

- Exercise

- Quit alcohol & cigarettes

- Subscribe to a body fat reduction plan in an esthetics clinic

- My challenges

- The work routine

- People's indifference

- Frustration

I hope you learned to recognize challenges you may encounter as well, I also hope now you know of some methods you could use to succeed, and some benefits of weight loss.

GNC pills:

GNC Pro Performance AMP Ripped Vitapak Program Supplement, 30 Count:

GNC Pro Performance AMP Women's Ripped Vitapak Program Supplement, 30 Count:

GNC Pro Performance AMP Men's Ripped Vitapak Program Supplement, 30 Count:

Success story: Karol's weight loss

Now, I want to show you Karol's weight loss story. Weight loss and staying healthy can change your life, and she is yet a clear and inspirational example for all of us.

She is married with two kids in elementary school, and from now on, she is a new friend of mine. Please read the interview I had with her. It is worth it.

Me: *Karol, what made you start a weight loss plan?*

Karol: *I started about three years ago. At that time, I felt really depressed, I had tried to lose weight before several times unsuccessfully, so I had become resigned that I was never going to change. Fortunately, my husband motivated me to lose weight by buying me a weight loss treatment with Xenical for two months, which I found very appealing and decided to give it a try.*

Me: *What has been the most difficult aspect of this process?*

Karol: *Persistence has been the most difficult side of this. It has been three years since that happened. I quit two years ago for around 8 months because back then I started working, and I was putting the exhaustion of work as an excuse to stop my plan, then I restarted as I was starting to gradually gain weight once again. Also, I believe my coworkers did not encourage me to stay on track whatsoever.*

Me: *What has been the most gratifying aspect(s)?*

Karol: *To be honest, being able to find clothes in all stores. Before, I had to ask in every store I saw a piece of clothing I liked what the largest size they had was, and I remember that was very frustrating.*

Also, being able to walk and run with ease. Before, I could not walk for a block without feeling really exhausted and almost fainting.

Me: *Now, do you know how many pounds you have lost so far, and for over what period of time?*

Karol: *Yes, I have lost 101 lbs so far over the past three years.*

However, I still want to lose 25 more lbs; that is my ultimate challenge at this moment.

Then, Karol smiles and asks me if I want to see photos of her three years ago before she started her weight-loss plan, to which I said yes. Let me tell you the photos are very impressive as the person displaying looks like another woman. Just picture a person with morbid obesity, and you will get the idea.

Me: *How did you feel before starting this process?*

Karol: *I used to feel really sad, back then I was taking care of my children and the house the whole day and my energy levels were too low. Moreover, I remember I used to believe that failures in my relationships with previous boyfriends I had were caused by me being overweight. I used to cry a lot every day.*

Me: *on the other hand, how do you feel now?*

Karol´s eyes turn watery, yet she still smiles.

Karol: *Happy, I believe when people say being overweight that they are happy with themselves is a lie. In my case, I never felt happy. Also, I feel with a lot more energy, and my mind is sharper.*

Me: *Karol, what would you recommend to people who are thinking about or have already decided to start a weight loss plan?*

Karol: *I would tell them to be persistent, and that the decision is within every one of us, that if you are not determined to lose weight and stay healthy no one else is going to make it happen. You need to be determined and persistent.*

Me: *So, would you say persistence is important in this process?*

Karol: *I am convinced persistence is essential.*

Me: *Can you tell us what you do when you feel like giving up? Do you use a technique in particular?*

Karol: *Whenever I feel down, because let me tell you, some days I wake up, and I do not feel like watching my diet; I rather feel like I want to eat that plate with anything I want. So, what I do is think that I do not want to be like before, I used to feel so bad. I remember how I was back then, and I tell myself I do not want to be that person again.*

Also, whenever I feel anxiety, I eat fruit as a snack, and that calms me down.

Me: *How do you see now the importance of taking care of yourself and health in general?*

K: *It is now a key issue for me. In the past, I did not give it the importance it requires, even after I saw my father died from diabetes.*

Me: *Finally, please tell us what did you exactly do to lose 100 pounds?*

K: *I ate and still eat healthily. For me, that meant to cut down the bread, and sodas, both of which I used to love. I started to eat vegetables and fruits, drink plenty of water instead of sodas. I hit the gym every week with my husband. This year, I became a vegetarian, and I started running, and I now feel more energized than last year.*

The interview ends here, we say goodbye and wish each other luck with our present weight loss challenges. As I head home, I feel so motivated to stay on track as I still am not finished with my weight loss yet. I still have 12 more lbs to go. But talking to a person like Karol, who has lost more than 100 lbs, has opened my eyes to the power that lies within every one of us.

WHAT I LEARNED FROM KAROL´S STORY

I liked her strong determination. Even though she admitted that she had stopped her plan for about eight months, she started back up afterwards. She was also extremely humble and honest about her experiences. I learned from her that the decision on losing weight is absolutely personal. No one else can win this fight for us, the only hero you can look up to is the person you see whenever you face a mirror.

I liked how she changed her view on life altogether with this experience. She said that she did not care about her health before, but finally she changed her views shifted.

Trust me here, it is so satisfactory see the healthy person she is now, and see that she has gained confidence, and overall, happiness. That is what Karol irradiates all over.

Now, please take a moment in this part of the book and reflect on what you can apply for to your own life from her testimony, please position your thoughts positively.

Short reminder on some of the perks of losing weight

- Higher energy levels.
- Satisfaction to achieve your goal.
- Being healthier.

In the next chapter, I am going to cover a method that can help you stay focused and succeed in your weight loss process.

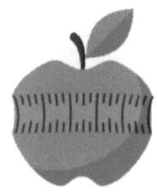

THE SEINFELD METHOD

Now, I would love to introduce you to the Seinfeld Method. This method –or strategy- is a great way to achieve goals and also improve ourselves along the way.

The story has to do with a famous person you probably know, Jerry Seinfeld, one of the most successful actors, comedians, writers, and producers. Widely known as the creator of the huge 90s show "Seinfeld", alongside Larry David. In 2002, TV Guide named Seinfeld the greatest television program of all time, among another large number of awards the show has received throughout its existence.

Please pay attention to this story. A software developer named Brad Isaac was doing open mic nights as a comic, and once he encountered and had a chance to speak with Jerry Seinfeld one of these nights. He went on and asked Mr. Seinfeld if he had any tips for a young comic…This is how Brad Isaacs tells the rest of the story:

"He revealed a unique calendar system he uses to pressure himself to write. Here's how it works.

He told me to get a big wall calendar that has a whole year on one page and hang it on a prominent wall. The next step was to get a big red magic marker.

He said for each day that I do my task of writing; I get to put a big red X over that day. "After a few days you'll have a chain. Just keep at it and the chain will grow longer every day. You'll like seeing that chain, especially when you get a few weeks under your belt. Your only job next is to not break the chain."

"Don't break the chain," he said again for emphasis.

Over the years, I've used his technique in many different areas. I've used it for exercise, to learn programming, to learn network administration, to build successful websites and build successful businesses.

It works because it isn't the one-shot pushes that get us where we want to go, it is the consistent daily action that builds extraordinary outcomes. You may have heard "inch by inch anything's a cinch." Inch by inch does work if you can move an inch every day."

You get me. Like I mentioned in previous parts of this book, being persistent and consistent is key to take ourselves where we want to go in life. Weight loss is a great goal to follow this strategy. The great lesson I get from Mr. Seinfeld´s method is that every bit of action grows over time in the path to achieving our goal.

Also, I also learned the task needing to be one are achievable. Not too simple, as you need to make progress with it, not too hard, as you need to be able to complete it on a daily basis.

There are many examples that can be related to persistence. I remember seeing this girl on YouTube, who danced every day for 365 days and recorded it progressively. When you see her on day one, she is not good, I mean, you can see she struggles to follow the choreography of the song at her apartment.

Little by little, she becomes better. Finally, on day 365, you can see she is dancing on a subway station with people watching and more importantly, she dances great! We all have that power within us.

Let me give you an example that can be applied to our goal at this time. You and I want to lose weight. So, we could make this daily task be to work out 15 minutes, or cut down sugar intake today. Then cross it out the calendar.

I have created a calendar myself to follow this exercise for this year and years to come. Would you like to try this strategy for yourself? Guess what. I have a gift for you. Please click below these lines where you can find a link to download a calendar to follow through this exercise. My suggestion is to put this calendar in a visible place to remind you of it. And remember, don't break the chain!

How to Lose Weight Fast

2015

January
Su	Mo	Tu	We	Th	Fr	Sa
				1	2	3
4	5	6	7	8	9	10
11	12	13	14	15	16	17
18	19	20	21	22	23	24
25	26	27	28	29	30	31

February
Su	Mo	Tu	We	Th	Fr	Sa
1	2	3	4	5	6	7
8	9	10	11	12	13	14
15	16	17	18	19	20	21
22	23	24	25	26	27	28

March
Su	Mo	Tu	We	Th	Fr	Sa
1	2	3	4	5	6	7
8	9	10	11	12	13	14
15	16	17	18	19	20	21
22	23	24	25	26	27	28
29	30	31				

April
Su	Mo	Tu	We	Th	Fr	Sa
			1	2	3	4
5	6	7	8	9	10	11
12	13	14	15	16	17	18
19	20	21	22	23	24	25
26	27	28	29	30		

May
Su	Mo	Tu	We	Th	Fr	Sa
					1	2
3	4	5	6	7	8	9
10	11	12	13	14	15	16
17	18	19	20	21	22	23
24	25	26	27	28	29	30
31						

June
Su	Mo	Tu	We	Th	Fr	Sa
	1	2	3	4	5	6
7	8	9	10	11	12	13
14	15	16	17	18	19	20
21	22	23	24	25	26	27
28	29	30				

July
Su	Mo	Tu	We	Th	Fr	Sa
			1	2	3	4
5	6	7	8	9	10	11
12	13	14	15	16	17	18
19	20	21	22	23	24	25
26	27	28	29	30	31	

August
Su	Mo	Tu	We	Th	Fr	Sa
						1
2	3	4	5	6	7	8
9	10	11	12	13	14	15
16	17	18	19	20	21	22
23	24	25	26	27	28	29
30	31					

September
Su	Mo	Tu	We	Th	Fr	Sa
		1	2	3	4	5
6	7	8	9	10	11	12
13	14	15	16	17	18	19
20	21	22	23	24	25	26
27	28	29	30			

October
Su	Mo	Tu	We	Th	Fr	Sa
				1	2	3
4	5	6	7	8	9	10
11	12	13	14	15	16	17
18	19	20	21	22	23	24
25	26	27	28	29	30	31

November
Su	Mo	Tu	We	Th	Fr	Sa
1	2	3	4	5	6	7
8	9	10	11	12	13	14
15	16	17	18	19	20	21
22	23	24	25	26	27	28
29	30					

December
Su	Mo	Tu	We	Th	Fr	Sa
		1	2	3	4	5
6	7	8	9	10	11	12
13	14	15	16	17	18	19
20	21	22	23	24	25	26
27	28	29	30	31		

Here is an online version too in case you do not want to print this out: https://goo.gl/KxvzQm

More on Jerry Seinfeld's Productivity Secret: http://goo.gl/Ccj7PF

More on the girl who learned to dance in a year: https://goo.gl/deVvtP

ELIMINATE HALF WORK

I would like you to please take a moment to think about this…How often do we find ourselves doing something important when a trivial distraction gets underway? Say you are in the middle of your workout, when suddenly you hear your phone ringing because of a Facebook notification. Here is yet another example.

You are preparing to cook your meal(s), when by chance you get an email from a guy who put you on their mailing list to sell you a product.

Such distractions are now so common for us that they go by every day unnoticed. They can do so much harm to our dreams and ambitions. When was the time we started getting distracted by so many fronts? I would say about ten years ago.

These distractions keep you away from a task that can make your day more productive, and as in the examples above, this applies to your weight loss efforts. My suggestion is that you turn off all gadgets that give these automatic updates or notifications while you are busy working out, cooking your meal, and so on. It may be difficult at first, but I know from experience this practice is of great support.

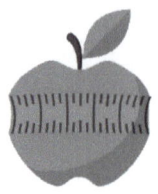

BONUS CONTENT

I want to give you an extra tip: Foods that help you burn calories & fat

These foods are going to help you lose weight. I have tried 4 of them, and they deliver.

Whole grains: Your body burns calories just to break down these grains. But how do I find whole grains? You can get brown rice, or whole oats.

Lean meats: A great source of protein. Skinless chicken breasts and turkey cutlets make the cut in this category.

Low-fat dairy products: Low-fat milk, low-fat yogurt. Stay away from sugars that may be added into these products (please read labels).

Green tea: Loaded with antioxidants and nutrients, green tea boosts metabolism and increases fat burning.

Lentils: These are rich in protein and loaded with soluble fiber.

Hot peppers: The component found in hot peppers called DCT (dihydrocapsiate) can help you burn a few extra calories and a bit more fat.

Best weight loss apps

Guys, technology can help us to stay on track with our weight loss and health along the way. I know I criticized distractions from technology, but I trust you can make good use of these apps and stay on track by now through persistence.

Let me introduce you to the best weight loss apps in the market at this moment: Follow this link http://goo.gl/R4IuBi

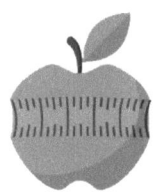

HOW PERSISTENCE APPLIES TO OTHER AREAS IN LIFE

Persistence means to persist, to keep going despite obstacles or setbacks, to continue moving forward no matter what.

You can look at almost any successful person in History, and they definitely could testify persistence was key to get to where they wanted to be.

J.K Rowling, the author of *Harry Potter*, her manuscript of the first Harry Potter, was initially rejected twelve times before it was finally given the green light.

The Beatles: They were rejected by many record labels. In a famous rejection, the label said, *"guitar groups are on the way out"* and *"the Beatles have no future in show business"*.

Vincent Van Gogh: He only sold one painting in his lifetime! Despite that he kept painting and finished over 800 pieces. Now everyone wants to buy them.

And the list goes on. I suggest you do this exercise: Think about two or three people you admire and you consider they achieved success by their own means. Then ask yourself: what did it take them to succeed? You will certainly find at some point they had to be persistent. There is no way to skip it.

Here are yet more stories of people I like and how they had to overcome obstacles, what they did to overcome them. Here are some of them.

Albert Einstein: He didn't speak till he was four and didn't read till seven. His parents and teachers thought he was mentally handicapped. He only turned out to win a Nobel prize and be the face of modern physics.

Colonel Sanders: The founder of KFC. He started his dream at 65 years old! He got a social security check for only $105 and was mad. Instead of complaining he did something about it.

He thought restaurant owners would love his fried chicken recipe, use it, sales would increase, and he'd get a percentage of it. He drove around the country knocking on doors, sleeping in his car, wearing his white suit until he got a "Yes".

Tim Ferris: The man behind the 4 Hour Workweek book, who changed how many people view work and life, was rejected by 26 publishers before one gave him a chance.

Persistence.

The good side of the story, what I want you to get from this chapter is that we all can be like these people.

What do we need? We need to commit to our goals no matter what setbacks may come. That's all. Another word comes along persistence: Determination. As defined in the Merriam-Webster dictionary, determination is a quality that makes you continue trying to do or achieve something that is difficult.

As a conclusion to this chapter, I hope now you can see the persistence you get from your weight loss process can make you a better person in other areas of your life as well.

READ MORE ON "FAMOUS PEOPLE WHO FOUND SUCCESS DESPITE FAILURE": http://goo.gl/TPmQgV

HEALTH IS AN INVESTMENT WORTH MILLIONS

Most of us have heard experts inspiring us to invest in Real Estate; Real Estate can be a great investment. Other experts suggest we invest in a brand new car (which in my opinion, it is not an investment by definition, as it only drains your wallet each month with the monthly fees).

However, let me explain my point for this section of the book. I want you to change perspective you may have had of the idea of health before reading this. I hope this can work as yet another reason to keep you losing weight, and even stay healthy after your weight loss is satisfactory.

I believe we all need to see health as a great way of investment. Yes, we need to visualize every effort we make to be healthy as an investment in life, happiness. We can get even more years since what we do before we enter our 50s is a way to guarantee that our years into late adulthood and old ages will be better and longer.

We all want to be healthy in our old age, am in wrong? Well, we need to understand that every bit of effort we put to stay active since we are children accumulates in the way of a compound effect throughout the years for our benefit.

Also, when we invest in our health, we are investing in having a more productive life in our years as young adults too. It is also one more benefit as this can help us generate more money for ourselves, our families, and even for the world (have you ever considered that charity is a great gift you can offer when you become wealthy, if that is your path at some point?)

On the contrary, we need to be convinced that investing proactively in our health is going to help us save money. We would have had to use to pay for treatment and medicines if we get a disease later on in our lives.

As we all know, insurance and medical plans are not cheap; even if they were cheap, would you not prefer to avoid pain, suffering for you and your loved ones?

How many times do we spend money literally on things that can bring momentary pleasure instead of something that makes wellbeing a permanent asset? Many times. Most of us who live in the Western world belong to a consumerist society that is always pushing us to buy the car, gadget, and so on of the moment. Why not stop and use this money in health instead.

We take health for granted; especially I think when we are young. Health really is a gift, and chances are our bodies will wear out throughout the years if we do not exercise, eat healthy, stay active, and avoid smoking and alcohol. We need to come to the realization that if we don't take ownership of our health, a disease could take over your life.

Finally, I want to thank you for going on this journey together by reading my book, I hope now you are more convinced to lose weight, and to be a healthy you.

I want to close with a quote from a famous American poet:

The first wealth is health.

Ralph Waldo Emerson

DISCLAIMER

All attempts have been made to verify the information contained in this book but the author and publisher do not bear any responsibility for errors or omissions. Any perceived negative connotation of any individual, group, or company is purely unintentional. Furthermore, this book is intended as entertainment only and as such, any and all responsibility for actions taken upon reading this book lies with the reader alone and not with the author or publisher. This book is not intended as medical, legal, or business advice and the reader alone holds sole responsibility for any consequences of any actions taken after reading this book. Additionally, it is the reader's responsibility alone and not the author's or publisher's to ensure that all applicable laws and regulations for business practice are adhered to. Lastly, I sometimes utilize affiliate links in the content of this book and as such, if you make a purchase through these links, I will gain a small commission.

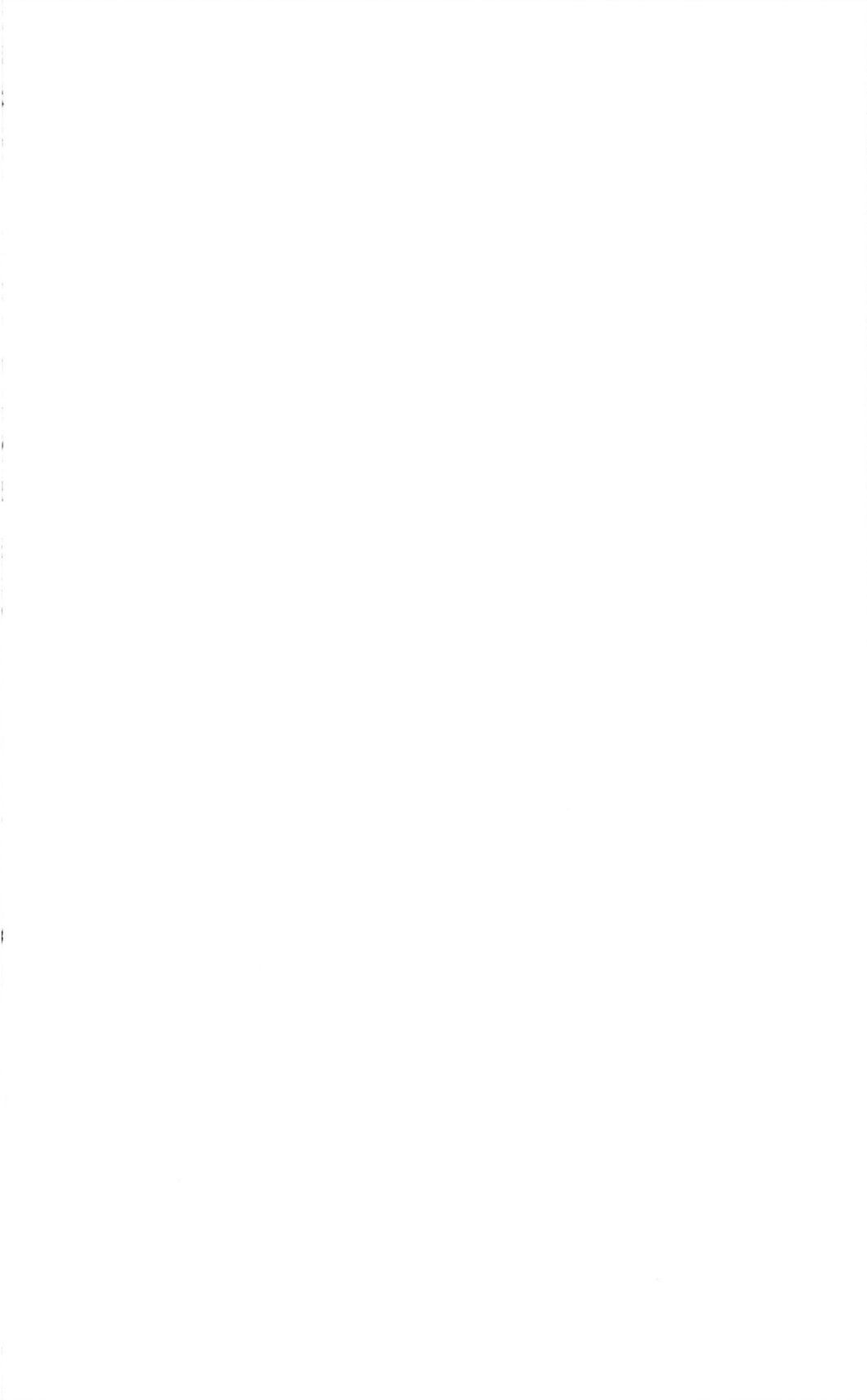